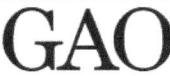

I0415810

February 2012

COMPARATIVE EFFECTIVENESS

Agency for Healthcare Research and Quality's Process for Awarding Recovery Act Funds and Disseminating Results

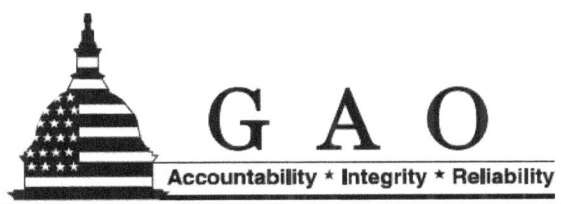

GAO-12-332

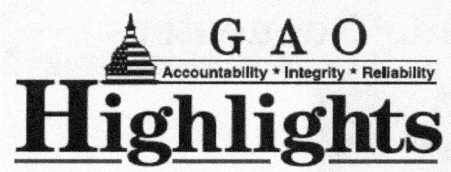

GAO
Accountability * Integrity * Reliability

Highlights

Highlights of GAO-12-332, a report to congressional requesters

COMPARATIVE EFFECTVENESS

Agency for Healthcare Research and Quality's Process for Awarding Recovery Act Funds and Disseminating Results

Why GAO Did This Study

The American Recovery and Reinvestment Act of 2009 (Recovery Act) provided $1.1 billion to the Department of Health and Human Services (HHS) for comparative effectiveness research (CER), which is research that compares different interventions and strategies to prevent, diagnose, treat, and monitor health conditions. Of this amount, HHS's Agency for Healthcare Research and Quality (AHRQ) received $474 million to support and disseminate the results of CER. GAO was asked to describe issues including the (1) process and criteria AHRQ used to award Recovery Act funds for CER, including steps to coordinate CER awards with other HHS entities in order to avoid unnecessary duplication of effort; and (2) plans AHRQ has for disseminating the results of CER it funded under the Recovery Act.

To address these objectives, GAO reviewed relevant documentation, including AHRQ's policies and procedures for selecting the recipients of grants; internal documents that describe the award of Recovery Act grants and contracts; and Recovery Act contractors' work plans. GAO also analyzed AHRQ data on the number and type of grants and contracts awarded Recovery Act CER funds. GAO interviewed AHRQ officials on the selection of Recovery Act CER grantees and contractors, including coordination with other HHS agencies that received Recovery Act CER funds, and the plans the agency has to disseminate the results of CER funded by the Recovery Act. AHRQ provided technical comments, which GAO incorporated as appropriate.

View GAO-12-332. For more information, contact Linda Kohn (202) 512-7114 or kohnl@gao.gov.

What GAO Found

AHRQ used its standard, competitive review processes and criteria to select the recipients of CER grants and contracts using Recovery Act funds. Specifically, to select the recipients of Recovery Act CER grants, AHRQ used its standard review process that includes peer review of grant applications, the development of funding recommendations by a team of senior officials within AHRQ, and final funding determination by the agency's director. As part of this process, AHRQ used its standard criteria to evaluate grant applications, as well as additional requirements that were specific to each funding opportunity. To select contractors who would receive Recovery Act funds, AHRQ used its standard contracting processes and criteria that are governed by the Federal Acquisition Regulation, which establishes uniform policies for acquisition of supplies and services by executive agencies, and the Public Health Service Act. These processes included an evaluation of all contract proposals using standard criteria adapted to the specific needs of each project. Between February 2009 and September 2010, AHRQ awarded $311 million of its $474 million in Recovery Act CER funds through 110 grants. AHRQ also awarded $161 million of its Recovery Act CER funding through 34 contracts. The contracts and grants AHRQ awarded supported both AHRQ's agency-specific and HHS's departmentwide CER priority areas. In an effort to avoid unnecessary duplication of CER awards, AHRQ participated in HHS working groups, developed a CER spending plan, and queried HHS databases to check for duplicative awards.

AHRQ's Recovery Act CER Funds ($474 million total)

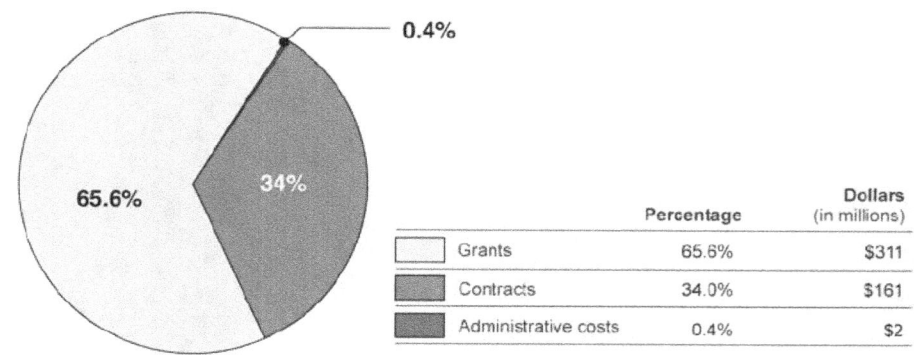

	Percentage	Dollars (in millions)
Grants	65.6%	$311
Contracts	34.0%	$161
Administrative costs	0.4%	$2

Source: GAO analysis of AHRQ data.

According to AHRQ officials, the agency plans to disseminate the results of Recovery Act-funded CER using a range of existing mechanisms. These mechanisms include written products, training programs, social media tools, and AHRQ's website. AHRQ is also developing additional strategies to disseminate CER results. AHRQ awarded four contracts using Recovery Act funds totaling approximately $42.3 million to promote innovative approaches for disseminating CER results. A variety of efforts are conducted under these contracts, including efforts to educate clinicians and develop regional dissemination offices.

_____ **United States Government Accountability Office**

Contents

Tables

Figures

Abbreviations

AHRQ	Agency for Healthcare Research and Quality
ASPE	Assistant Secretary for Planning and Evaluation
CER	comparative effectiveness research
CER-CIT	Comparative Effectiveness Research-Coordination and Implementation Team
COTR	contracting officer's technical representative
FAR	Federal Acquisition Regulation
FOA	funding opportunity announcement
GSA	General Services Administration
HHS	Department of Health and Human Services
MMA	Medicare Prescription Drug, Improvement, and Modernization Act of 2003
NIH	National Institutes of Health
OMB	Office of Management and Budget
PHSA	Public Health Service Act
PPACA	Patient Protection and Affordable Care Act
PCORI	Patient-Centered Outcomes Research Institute
PCORTF	Patient-Centered Outcomes Research Trust Fund
Recovery Act	American Recovery and Reinvestment Act of 2009
VHA	Veterans Health Administration

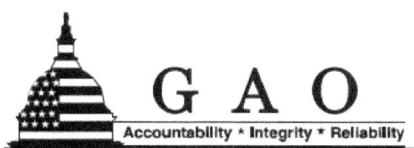

United States Government Accountability Office
Washington, DC 20548

February 29, 2012

The Honorable Fred Upton
Chairman
Committee on Energy and Commerce
House of Representatives

The Honorable Joe Barton
House of Representatives

Since the enactment of the Medicare Prescription Drug, Improvement, and Modernization Act of 2003 (MMA), the Agency for Healthcare Research and Quality (AHRQ), an agency within the Department of Health and Human Services (HHS), has been one of several federal agencies responsible for supporting and disseminating the results of comparative effectiveness research (CER).[1,2] CER is research that compares different interventions and strategies to prevent, diagnose, treat, and monitor health conditions. AHRQ has supported CER activities and disseminated results by awarding grants and contracts to research centers and academic organizations to carry out this work. These grantees and contractors review and synthesize scientific evidence through research reviews; generate new scientific evidence and analytical tools in original research reports; and compile research findings that are translated into formats for a variety of audiences. The results of CER can be used by both patients and clinicians to make health care decisions about which treatment or intervention may be most effective or beneficial for a given patient.[3]

Under the American Recovery and Reinvestment Act of 2009 (Recovery Act), AHRQ received significant funding to support and disseminate the results of CER. Specifically, while AHRQ's fiscal years 2009 and 2010

---

[1]This mission was assigned to AHRQ by the MMA. Pub. L. No. 108-173, § 1013, 117 Stat. 2066, 2438-41 (2003) (codified at 42 U.S.C. § 299b-7). Other federal agencies that conduct CER include the National Institutes of Health (NIH) and the Veterans Health Administration (VHA), a component of the Department of Veterans Affairs.

[2]AHRQ also refers to CER as patient-centered outcomes research.

[3]U.S. Department of Health and Human Services, *Federal Coordinating Council for Comparative Effectiveness Research: Report to the President and the Congress* (Washington, D.C.: June 30, 2009).

budgets for CER activities were $50 million and $21 million, respectively, the Recovery Act provided AHRQ with an additional $474 million for CER for this period—$300 million that was appropriated to AHRQ and $174 million that was appropriated to the HHS Office of the Secretary and allocated to AHRQ.[4] The Recovery Act, which was enacted on February 17, 2009, required that AHRQ obligate these funds by September 30, 2010.[5] AHRQ's $474 million in funding was part of $1.1 billion HHS received under the Recovery Act to support CER through its various agencies, including AHRQ and the National Institutes of Health (NIH).

The Patient Protection and Affordable Care Act (PPACA) gave AHRQ additional responsibilities related to CER—in particular, responsibilities related to the Patient-Centered Outcomes Research Institute (PCORI). PCORI is a nonprofit corporation established by PPACA to, among other things, improve the quality and relevance of CER, and disseminate the results of this research.[6] AHRQ is to help PCORI meet its mission in several ways, which include broadly disseminating the results of the research that PCORI conducts or funds;[7] developing a publicly available

---

[4]The act appropriated $400 million to the HHS Office of the Secretary to distribute to HHS agencies to carry out CER; the Office of the Secretary allocated $174 million of these funds to AHRQ. HHS agencies that received a portion of these funds awarded contracts and grants through internal agency processes to carry out specific CER projects in four priority areas. Other HHS agencies that received a portion of these funds include the Centers for Medicare & Medicaid Services, the Food and Drug Administration, NIH, and the Centers for Disease Control and Prevention.

[5]An obligation is a definite commitment that creates a legal liability of the government that will give rise to a payment immediately or in the future. An agency incurs an obligation when it awards a grant or contract.

[6]PPACA authorized the establishment of PCORI, a nonprofit corporation, to assist patients, clinicians, purchasers, and policymakers in making informed health decisions by advancing the quality and relevance of evidence concerning the manner in which diseases, disorders, and other health conditions can effectively and appropriately be prevented, diagnosed, treated, monitored, and managed through research and evidence synthesis that considers variations in subpopulations and dissemination of research findings in several areas. PCORI's duties include identifying research priorities, establishing a research project agenda, and carrying out that agenda using a variety of methodological approaches. PPACA required the Comptroller General of the United States to appoint 19 members to PCORI's Board of Governors, which he did in September 2010. See Pub. L. No. 111-148, §§ 6301(a), 10602, 124 Stat. 119, 727-38, 1005 (2010) (to be codified at 42 U.S.C. § 1320e).

[7]Pub. L. No. 111-148, § 6301(b), 124 Stat. 119, 738-40 (2010) (to be codified at 42 U.S.C. § 299b-37).

database for this research; and promoting the incorporation of CER findings into health information technology systems that support clinical decision making.[8]

In June 2011, we provided information to congressional committees on HHS's use of CER funds that were available under the Recovery Act and PPACA.[9] You have also asked that we report on AHRQ's procedures for awarding Recovery Act CER funds and AHRQ's plans to address the various new responsibilities established for it by PPACA as they relate to PCORI. In this report, we describe (1) the process and criteria AHRQ used to award Recovery Act funds for CER, including steps to coordinate these awards with other HHS entities in order to avoid unnecessary duplication of effort; (2) the plans AHRQ has for disseminating the results of CER it funded under the Recovery Act; and (3) the steps AHRQ has taken to perform its roles and responsibilities related to PCORI under PPACA.

Scope and Methodology

To describe the process and criteria AHRQ used to award its $474 million in Recovery Act CER funds, we reviewed relevant statutes as well as documentation on the process and criteria AHRQ uses to (1) determine the scientific and technical merit of grant applications and contract proposals, and (2) select grant recipients and contractors. We reviewed spending plans, which outline AHRQ's and HHS's plans for spending Recovery Act funds. We also reviewed summary statements that describe AHRQ's process for selecting grantees and contractors to be awarded Recovery Act funds. In addition, we reviewed AHRQ's Management Operations Manual, the agency's written guidance that provides policies and procedures for selecting grant recipients.[10] We interviewed AHRQ and other HHS officials to learn about the processes and criteria they used to select the grantees and contractors that received awards funded

---

[8]See Pub. L. No. 111-148, §§ 6301(a), (b), 10602, 124 Stat. 119, 727-47, 1005 (2010) (to be codified at 42 U.S.C. §§ 299b-37, 1320e).

[9]GAO, *HHS Research Awards: Use of Recovery Act and Patient Protection and Affordable Care Act Funds for Comparative Effectiveness Research*, GAO-11-712R (Washington, D.C.: June 14, 2011).

[10]The sections of AHRQ's Management Operations Manual that provide policies and procedures for selecting the recipients of grants are primarily composed of HHS's Awarding Agency Grants Administration Manual, which is HHS's grant application manual.

with the $474 million in Recovery Act CER funds and to coordinate these awards with other HHS agencies that also received Recovery Act CER funds. Because NIH also received Recovery Act CER funds, we conducted interviews with NIH officials to confirm the methods and processes used by AHRQ to coordinate funding opportunity announcements (FOA), contract solicitations, and awards with NIH in an effort to prevent the unnecessary duplication of effort in awarding Recovery Act CER funds.[11] Finally, we obtained data from AHRQ on the number and type of awards made between February 2009 and September 2010 using the $474 million in Recovery Act CER funds. We relied on Recovery Act award data provided by AHRQ and did not audit the reported data. To determine whether AHRQ and the Office of the Secretary's Recovery Act CER award data were sufficiently reliable for our analyses, we conducted a reliability assessment of the data we used by reviewing existing information about the data, conducting quality control checks, and interviewing agency officials knowledgeable about the data. We determined that the data were sufficiently reliable for the purposes of this report.

To describe AHRQ's plans to disseminate results from CER funded with Recovery Act funds, we reviewed the Recovery Act and other relevant statutes to determine AHRQ's responsibilities for disseminating CER. We reviewed agency documents, including AHRQ contractors' work plans describing specific goals and activities; AHRQ's general publications, including reports and guides posted on AHRQ's website and electronic newsletters; and samples of AHRQ's CER, including original research reports, treatment guides, and slide presentations used for educating clinicians. We also interviewed AHRQ officials and a contractor to understand how the agency plans to disseminate the results of CER funded with Recovery Act funds and to obtain information on plans AHRQ has for assessing the effectiveness of its dissemination efforts.

To describe the steps AHRQ has taken to fulfill its roles and responsibilities related to PCORI under PPACA, we reviewed provisions in PPACA to identify these roles and responsibilities, which include to broadly disseminate CER findings to various audiences; develop a

---

[11]FOAs and contract solicitations announce an agency's intent to fund research or other work through a grant or contract, respectively. FOAs and solicitations include a description of the research or work to be performed and criteria against which applicants will be considered.

publicly available database to collect evidence and research; and promote the timely incorporation of CER findings into health information technology systems that support clinical decision making.[12] While AHRQ is required to conduct a number of activities under PPACA, we focused our review on those activities that are related to PCORI. We also reviewed AHRQ's PPACA spending plan for fiscal years 2011 and 2012, which describes the agency's plans for using funds made available by PPACA, as well as PCORI presentation materials and meeting reports. We also conducted interviews with AHRQ officials to determine the steps the agency has taken to meet its responsibilities related to PCORI under PPACA.

We conducted this performance audit from February 2011 to February 2012 in accordance with generally accepted government auditing standards. Those standards require that we plan and perform the audit to obtain sufficient, appropriate evidence to provide a reasonable basis for our findings and conclusions based on our audit objectives. We believe that the evidence obtained provides a reasonable basis for our findings and conclusions based on our audit objectives.

Background

AHRQ supports CER by awarding grants and contracts to entities in order to conduct CER and perform related activities, such as the dissemination of CER results.[13] As 1 of 12 agencies within HHS, AHRQ's overarching mission is to improve the quality, safety, efficiency, and effectiveness of health care for all Americans. (For more information on AHRQ's mission, research, priorities, and budget, see app. I.)

CER and the Recovery Act

The Recovery Act provided a significant amount of funding for AHRQ to conduct CER activities. (See table 1.)

---

[12]See Pub. L. No. 111-148, §§ 6301(a), (b), 10602, 124 Stat. 119, 727-47, 1005 (2010) (to be codified at 42 U.S.C. §§ 299b-37, 1320e).

[13]The term dissemination refers to developing and distributing messages that are derived from CER for target audiences such as clinicians, consumers, or policymakers in order to inform health care delivery or practice.

Table 1: AHRQ's Funding for CER Activities, Fiscal Years 2007 through 2011

Fiscal year	Funding from annual appropriations (in millions)[a]	Funding from other appropriations (in millions)
2007	$15.0	
2008	30.0	
2009	50.0	$474.0[b]
2010	21.0	
2011	21.0	$8.0[c]

Source: AHRQ.

[a]Language in committee reports accompanying annual appropriations acts directs AHRQ to use specified amounts for CER activities from a lump sum appropriation.

[b]The Recovery Act was enacted on February 17, 2009, and AHRQ received a total of $474 million for CER under the Recovery Act — $300 million that was appropriated to AHRQ and $174 million that was appropriated to the HHS Office of the Secretary and allocated to AHRQ. The Recovery Act required that these funds be obligated by September 30, 2010. An obligation is a definite commitment that creates a legal liability of the government that will give rise to a payment immediately or in the future.

[c]These funds were made available to AHRQ in fiscal year 2011 from the Patient-Centered Outcomes Research Trust Fund.

HHS developed departmentwide priorities for CER. (See table 2.) Of the total amount of $474 million in Recovery Act funds available to AHRQ for CER, $174 million of these funds were allocated to AHRQ by the Office of the Secretary and were used to support the HHS departmentwide priorities for CER.

Table 2: HHS Departmentwide Priority Areas for CER Funded by the Recovery Act

Priority area	Description
Data Infrastructure	Enhance existing data infrastructure and develop new databases, networks, and registries to support CER. Essential investments include longitudinal databases to link claims data for individual patients over a long period of time and patient registries that will prospectively collect clinical data on patients with specific diseases or on specific tests or procedures.
Dissemination, Translation, and Implementation	Ensure innovative strategies to invest in the dissemination and implementation of CER with the ultimate goal being improved health outcomes. Funded projects include efforts to advance the dissemination of CER to patients and providers; and dissemination and implementation efforts at the delivery system and community levels.
Research	Provide information on the relative strengths and weaknesses of various medical interventions.
Inventory and Evaluation	Catalogue CER activities and infrastructure in order to track investments in CER going forward.

Source: AHRQ.

AHRQ developed seven agency-specific CER priority areas to guide its spending of Recovery Act funds. (See table 3.) Of the total amount of $474 million in Recovery Act funds available to AHRQ for CER, $300 million of these funds were appropriated to the agency and, therefore, supported the agency's seven CER priority areas.

Table 3: AHRQ Priority Areas for CER Funded by the Recovery Act

Priority area	Description
Horizon Scanning	Identify new and emerging issues for CER investments and establish an approach to investigate and prioritize areas for investigation relevant to the 14 priority conditions that guide the Effective Health Care Program.[a]
Evidence Synthesis	Increase the number of CER reviews conducted by AHRQ's Evidence-based Practice Centers.
Evidence Gap Identification	Identify gaps in evidence research and prioritize needs for future reviews.
Translation and Dissemination	Expand the translation of findings on CER for different audiences, such as consumers, clinicians, and policymakers, and disseminate those findings.
Evidence Generation	Measure the effectiveness of treatments for priority conditions with a concentration in under-represented populations, including children, the elderly, and racial and ethnic minorities.
Training and Career Development	Enhance the research and methodological capacity for conducting and improving CER and the development of data sources and research infrastructure.
Community Forum	Formally engage stakeholders in CER efforts and develop a process for formal advice and guidance.

Source: AHRQ.

[a]These priority conditions are arthritis and nontraumatic joint disorders; cancer; cardiovascular disease, including stroke and hypertension; dementia, including Alzheimer's disease; depression and other mental health disorders; developmental delays, attention-deficit hyperactivity disorder, and autism; diabetes mellitus; functional limitations and disability; infectious diseases, including HIV/AIDS; obesity; peptic ulcer disease and dyspepsia; pregnancy, including preterm birth; pulmonary disease/asthma; and substance abuse.

CER and the Patient Protection and Affordable Care Act

The enactment of PPACA in 2010 gave AHRQ new roles and responsibilities related to disseminating CER and building capacity for research, and appropriated funds for carrying out these activities. Several of these responsibilities relate to work conducted by PCORI. Established in November 2010, PCORI was authorized to help coordinate CER at a national level by developing national priorities for CER and conducting and funding CER activities. PPACA directs AHRQ to broadly disseminate CER findings to physicians, other health care providers, patients, payers, and policymakers; develop a publicly available database to collect evidence and research; promote the timely incorporation of CER findings into health information technology systems that support clinical decision making; and establish a process for receiving feedback about the value of information disseminated by AHRQ.[14]

To fund this work, PPACA established the Patient-Centered Outcomes Research Trust Fund (PCORTF). The act specified that percentages of this trust fund be provided to the Secretary of HHS and AHRQ in each of fiscal years 2011 through 2019.[15] Specifically, AHRQ received $8 million from this trust fund in fiscal year 2011 and will receive $24 million in fiscal year 2012, representing 16 percent of the total amount appropriated to this trust fund in each of these fiscal years. In subsequent fiscal years, AHRQ will continue to receive 16 percent of the total amount appropriated to the trust fund, which will be based on the net revenues from fees on health insurance and self-insured plans, amounts transferred from the Medicare trust funds, and appropriations to PCORTF from the General Fund of the Treasury.

AHRQ's Standard Competitive Process for Selecting Grant Recipients

A portion of AHRQ's work, including its work related to CER, is conducted through grants awarded to research centers and academic organizations to fund research ideas developed by a grant applicant. Grant applications are submitted in response to publicly available FOAs, which announce AHRQ's intention to award research grants. AHRQ has established a standard competitive process that is governed by federal law to select grant recipients.[16] According to AHRQ officials, this multistep process includes: (1) an initial review of received applications; (2) preliminary scoring of applications; (3) review and final scoring of applications at a peer review panel meeting; (4) the development of preliminary funding recommendations; (5) review by a senior leadership team within AHRQ; and (6) a final determination of funding by the agency director.

[14]See Pub. L. No. 111-148, §§ 6301(a), (b), 10602, 124 Stat. 119, 727-47, 1005 (2010) (to be codified at 42 U.S.C. §§ 299b-37, 1320e).

[15]The trustee of PCORTF is to provide for the transfer from PCORTF of 20 percent of the amounts appropriated or credited to PCORTF for each of fiscal years 2011 through 2019 to the Secretary of HHS. Of the amounts transferred, the Secretary of HHS is to distribute 80 percent to AHRQ and 20 percent to the Secretary of HHS. See 26 U.S.C. § 9511.

[16]AHRQ's process for selecting grant recipients is governed by the Public Health Service Act (PHSA) and implementing regulations, which require the use of peer review for grant applications to ensure fair, competent, and objective assessment of their scientific and technical merit. See 42 U.S.C.§ 299c-1; 42 C.F.R. pt. 67, subpt. A.

To evaluate the grant applications it receives in response to FOAs, AHRQ's peer reviewers, most of whom are authorities in their respective fields and not government employees, use five standard core criteria to score and rank the applications. These five standard core criteria are (1) the significance in addressing an important problem; (2) the investigators' ability to carry out the research; (3) the originality or innovation of the project; (4) the development of an adequate research approach or framework; and (5) the scientific environment in which the applicant plans to conduct the research. Each FOA also contains criteria that are specific to the announcement. While these other specific criteria are not individually scored, they are used to evaluate the applications during the peer review panel meetings. (See fig. 1 for an overview of AHRQ's standard process for selecting grant recipients.)

Figure 1: AHRQ's Standard Competitive Process for Selecting Grant Recipients

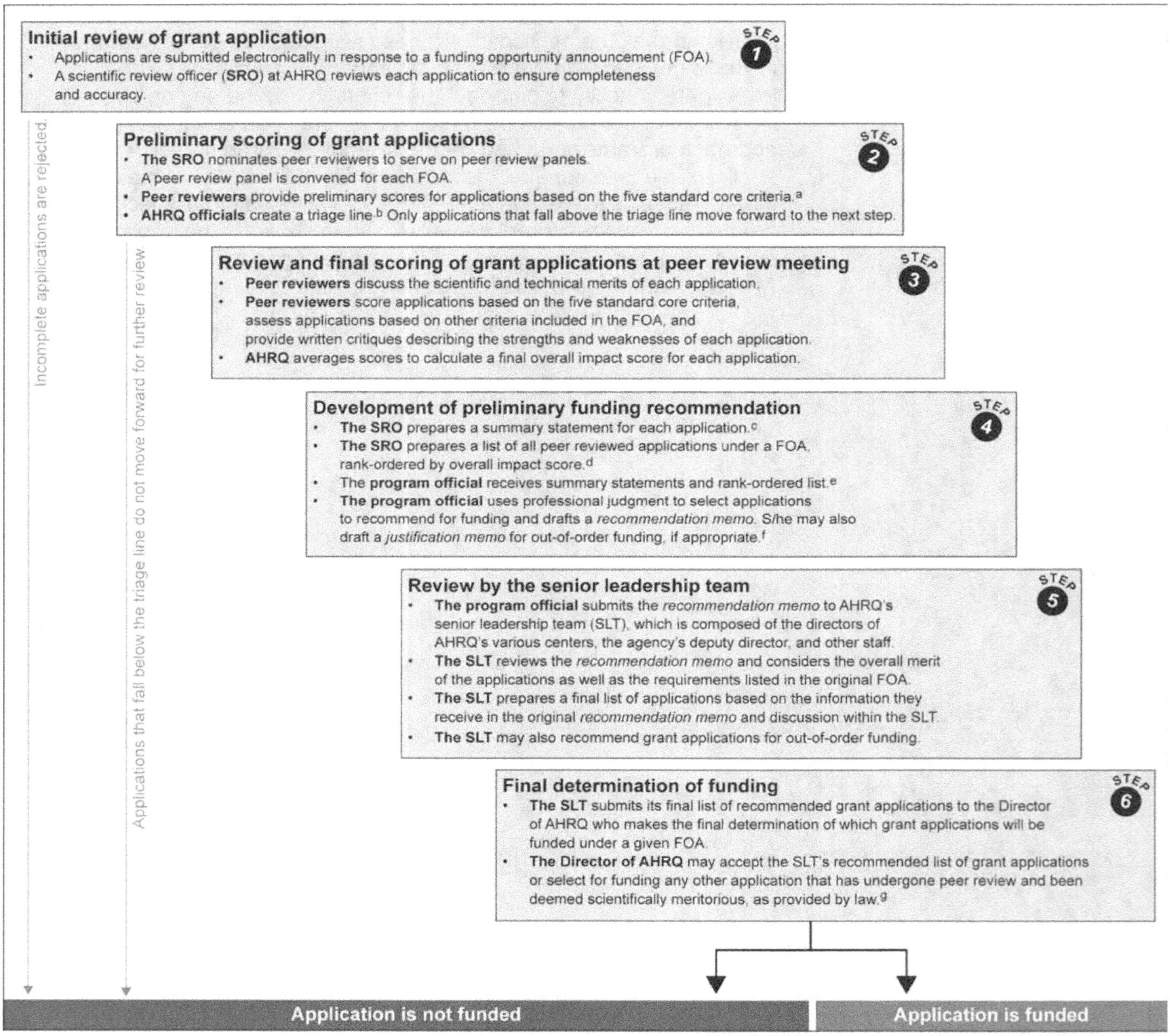

Initial review of grant application — STEP 1
- Applications are submitted electronically in response to a funding opportunity announcement (FOA).
- A scientific review officer (SRO) at AHRQ reviews each application to ensure completeness and accuracy.

Preliminary scoring of grant applications — STEP 2
- The SRO nominates peer reviewers to serve on peer review panels. A peer review panel is convened for each FOA.
- Peer reviewers provide preliminary scores for applications based on the five standard core criteria.[a]
- AHRQ officials create a triage line.[b] Only applications that fall above the triage line move forward to the next step.

Review and final scoring of grant applications at peer review meeting — STEP 3
- Peer reviewers discuss the scientific and technical merits of each application.
- Peer reviewers score applications based on the five standard core criteria, assess applications based on other criteria included in the FOA, and provide written critiques describing the strengths and weaknesses of each application.
- AHRQ averages scores to calculate a final overall impact score for each application.

Development of preliminary funding recommendation — STEP 4
- The SRO prepares a summary statement for each application.[c]
- The SRO prepares a list of all peer reviewed applications under a FOA, rank-ordered by overall impact score.[d]
- The program official receives summary statements and rank-ordered list.[e]
- The program official uses professional judgment to select applications to recommend for funding and drafts a *recommendation memo*. S/he may also draft a *justification memo* for out-of-order funding, if appropriate.[f]

Review by the senior leadership team — STEP 5
- The program official submits the *recommendation memo* to AHRQ's senior leadership team (SLT), which is composed of the directors of AHRQ's various centers, the agency's deputy director, and other staff.
- The SLT reviews the *recommendation memo* and considers the overall merit of the applications as well as the requirements listed in the original FOA.
- The SLT prepares a final list of applications based on the information they receive in the original *recommendation memo* and discussion within the SLT.
- The SLT may also recommend grant applications for out-of-order funding.

Final determination of funding — STEP 6
- The SLT submits its final list of recommended grant applications to the Director of AHRQ who makes the final determination of which grant applications will be funded under a given FOA.
- The Director of AHRQ may accept the SLT's recommended list of grant applications or select for funding any other application that has undergone peer review and been deemed scientifically meritorious, as provided by law.[g]

Incomplete applications are rejected

Applications that fall below the triage line do not move forward for further review

Application is not funded | **Application is funded**

Source: GAO analysis of AHRQ documents and interviews with AHRQ officials.

[a]Each application is reviewed by three peer reviewers who assign preliminary scores.

GAO-12-332 AHRQ Comparative Effectiveness Research

[b]AHRQ establishes a minimum score, or triage line, that the grant applications must receive in order to proceed to the next level of peer review. The triage line is established so that the number of applications that fall above the triage line can be reasonably reviewed by the peer review panel at the next stage; the poorest-scoring 50 percent to 60 percent of applications are eliminated; or the peer review panel can review about three times the number of applications AHRQ anticipates funding under a given FOA.

[c]The summary statement includes peer reviewers' written critiques, budget recommendations, administrative notes, and the final overall impact score for the application.

[d]"Rank order" refers to the relative position of an application among a listing of applications that have undergone peer review. The listing of applications is ranked in the order of the overall impact score calculated during the peer review process, from most to least meritorious.

[e]The program official is the AHRQ official responsible for the program area of the FOA.

[f]"Out-of-order funding" occurs when applications are funded out of rank order (i.e., not in accordance with the rank order of most-meritorious to least-meritorious based on the overall impact scores calculated during the peer review process). A program official may recommend and the agency may ultimately decide to make out-of-order funding decisions for a number of reasons including the need to address important agency research priorities, avoid duplication, or meet specific requirements in the original FOA that the more meritorious applications cannot meet. The Director of AHRQ makes the final determination to fund grant applications, including any out-of-order funding decisions. For any out-of-order funding decision, a justification memo is prepared to provide written justification of why out-of-order funding is being recommended.

[g]The Director of AHRQ may not approve an application for funding unless the application has been recommended for approval by a peer review group. 42 U.S.C. § 299c-1(b); 42 C.F.R. § 67.16(b) .

AHRQ's Standard Competitive Processes for Awarding Contracts

AHRQ uses a separate competitive process to award contracts, which fund specific activities defined by AHRQ. This process for selecting contract proposals for award is governed by the Federal Acquisition Regulation (FAR)[17] and the Public Health Service Act (PHSA) and implementing regulations.[18] The advertising of available contracting opportunities, which occurs through different types of solicitations, varies depending on the type of contracting mechanism used. AHRQ generally uses three types of contracting mechanisms.

- **Stand-alone contracts**. This contracting vehicle involves the issuance of new, stand-alone contracts. Proposals are submitted in response to publicly-available solicitations referred to as requests for proposals. A request for proposals details the specific tasks or ideas that an agency needs a contractor to fulfill, such as delivery of a certain service or research of a clearly defined topic.

---

[17]48 C.F.R. ch. 1. The FAR establishes uniform policies for acquisition of supplies and services by executive agencies. Agency acquisition regulations may implement or supplement the FAR.

[18]The PHSA and implementing regulations require the use of peer review of contract proposals. See 42 U.S.C. § 299c-1; 42 C.F.R. pt. 67, subpt. B.

- **Task orders**. This contracting vehicle involves issuing task orders under an existing, master contract, thereby giving a contractor a new task to perform. Proposals are submitted in response to solicitations called requests for task orders, which are issued to contractors already awarded contracts by the agency.

- **General Services Administration (GSA)-schedule task orders**. This contracting vehicle involves the use of contracts that have been awarded by GSA for governmentwide use. GSA-schedule task orders are issued under existing master contracts awarded by GSA. These task orders are solicited through a request for quote solicitation that is competed among these contractors.

Upon receiving proposals in response to a solicitation, AHRQ typically evaluates contract proposals for award using standard contracting procedures and criteria, which are governed by the FAR and the PHSA and implementing regulations. A technical review panel of agency officials and external experts evaluates each proposal submitted in response to a solicitation against standard criteria that are tailored to the specific needs of each solicitation. These criteria include (1) demonstrated knowledge and understanding of the contract requirements; (2) the proposed approach to address tasks and subtasks listed in the proposal; (3) the qualifications and experience of key management personnel, such as the project director and project manager; (4) the potential contractor's ability to meet the project's milestones; (5) the facility, equipment, and space available to support the project goals and objectives; and (6) the past performance of the potential contractor using information from references or other government customers. Based on this evaluation of each proposal's scientific and technical merit and cost, the review panel, along with the contracting officer's technical representative (COTR),[19] identifies the entity they believe should be awarded the contract and forwards the recommendation to the contracting officer, the federal official who has

---

[19]A COTR is a government official who is designated by the agency's contracting officer to assist in the technical monitoring or administration of a contract.

authority to enter into a contract.[20] The contracting officer reviews the recommendation and makes a final award decision.[21]

AHRQ Used Standard Competitive Processes and Criteria and Coordinated within HHS to Make Recovery Act Awards

AHRQ used its standard, competitive review process and criteria to select grant recipients and award 110 Recovery Act-funded CER grants, totaling approximately $311 million. In addition, AHRQ primarily used its standard contracting processes and criteria to select contract proposals and enter into 34 contracts for CER using Recovery Act funding, totaling approximately $161 million. AHRQ also took several steps to coordinate with other HHS agencies when soliciting and awarding CER grants and contracts.

AHRQ Used Its Standard Competitive Review Process and Criteria to Select Grant Recipients and Award 110 CER Grants

Between February 2009 and September 2010, AHRQ used its standard, competitive grant review process to select grant recipients and ultimately award 110 CER grants using approximately $311 million in Recovery Act CER funds. Specifically, AHRQ used its standard process for selecting grantees, which includes an initial review and preliminary scoring of applications; review and final scoring of applications at peer review panel meetings; development of preliminary funding recommendations; review of funding recommendations by a senior leadership team within AHRQ; and a final determination of funding by the agency director.

As part of the standard process AHRQ used to select the recipients of Recovery Act-funded CER grants, peer reviewers used the agency's standard core criteria to score and subsequently rank the applications for this funding. In addition to its core criteria, AHRQ also used other criteria in its process of selecting recipients of Recovery Act CER grants. These other criteria were specific to each FOA and often varied depending on the CER study requested under that announcement. These other criteria may be used to assess, for example, a grant application in terms of the

---

[20]Contracting officers are responsible for ensuring performance of all necessary actions for effective contracting. Contracting officers enter into, administer, and terminate contracts.

[21]The contracting officer may not award a contract unless the proposal has been recommended for approval by the review panel. See 42 U.S.C. § 299c-1(b); 42 C.F.R. § 67.103.

adequacy of the protection afforded human subjects; the inclusion of certain priority populations in the study;[22] the extent to which privacy and security issues have been addressed; the partnerships that the applicant has with the proposed population; and the degree of responsiveness in addressing the purpose and objective of the FOA. AHRQ officials told us that the agency's peer reviewers, program officials, and members of the senior leadership team used both standard core criteria and other criteria outlined in the FOAs to determine which grant applications should be recommended to the Director of AHRQ for funding.

AHRQ issued 14 FOAs for Recovery Act CER grant opportunities. Using its grant review process and criteria, AHRQ received 536 grant applications and awarded 110 CER grants between February 2009 and September 2010, totaling approximately $311 million.[23,24] The roughly $311 million in grants AHRQ awarded supported HHS's departmentwide and AHRQ's agency-specific CER priorities. (See fig. 2 and app. II for more information on the award of AHRQ's CER grants with Recovery Act funds.)

---

[22]AHRQ is directed to conduct and support research with respect to health care for priority populations. These priority populations include low-income groups, women, the elderly, minorities, individuals with disabilities, and recipients of rural health care. See 42 U.S.C. § 299(c)(1) . For more information on AHRQ's priority populations, see http://www.ahrq.gov/populations/.

[23]The 14 FOAs issued and 110 CER grants awarded addressed projects in three of the four HHS-departmentwide CER priority areas and three of AHRQ's seven agency-specific CER priority areas. Some priority areas were supported by more than one FOA. AHRQ agency-specific and HHS departmentwide priority areas not supported with grants were supported through contracts.

[24]AHRQ made these awards by September 30, 2010, the end of the period in which the Recovery Act funds were available for obligation. See GAO-11-712R. AHRQ awarded an additional $161 million through contracts and spent approximately $2 million for administrative purposes.

Figure 2: Distribution of AHRQ's Recovery Act Funds for CER Grants, by Priority Area

AHRQ's CER priority areas ($200 million total)[a]

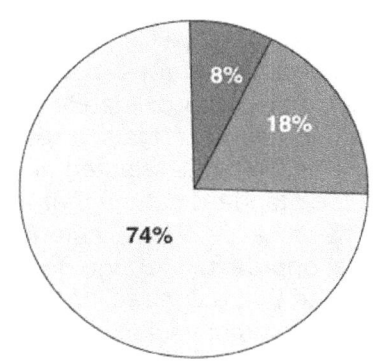

HHS's departmentwide CER priority areas ($111 million total)[b]

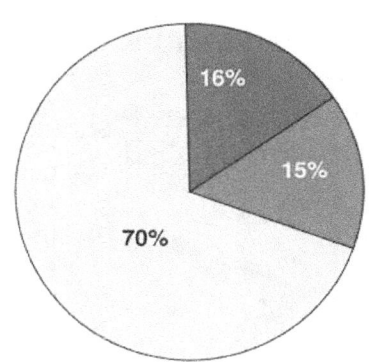

	Percentage[c]	Dollars (in millions)
Evidence Generation	74%	$148.8
Training and Development	8%	$15.4
Translation and Dissemination	18%	$35.7

	Percentage[c]	Dollars (in millions)
Data Infrastructure	70%	$77.4
Translation and Dissemination	15%	$16.2
Research	16%	$17.8

Source: GAO analysis of AHRQ data.

[a]AHRQ supported the remaining four CER priority areas through contracts.

[b]AHRQ supported the one remaining HHS departmentwide CER priority area through contracts.

[c]Percentages do not add up to 100 percent due to rounding.

For 55 of the 110 grants, the Director of AHRQ exercised her discretion to make out-of-order funding decisions.[25] An out-of-order funding decision occurs when grant applications are funded out of rank order; that is, they are not funded in accordance with the rank order of most-meritorious to least-meritorious overall impact scores calculated during the peer review process. Out-of-order funding decisions can be made for a number of reasons, including the need to address important agency research priorities, avoid duplication, or meet specific requirements in the original FOA that the more meritorious applicants cannot meet. Recommendations for out-of-order funding decisions are made by the

---

[25]The Director of AHRQ may not approve an application for funding unless the application has been recommended for approval by a peer review group. 42 U.S.C. § 299c-1(b); 42 C.F.R. § 67.16(b).

GAO-12-332 AHRQ Comparative Effectiveness Research

program official or senior leadership team, but the final decision to award grants is made by the Director of AHRQ.[26]

AHRQ Primarily Used Its Standard Competitive Contracting Process and Criteria to Award 34 CER Contracts

Between February 2009 and September 2010, AHRQ primarily used its standard competitive contracting process and criteria to select contract proposals and enter into 34 contracts using approximately $161 million in Recovery Act CER funds. According to AHRQ officials, a review panel, composed of external experts and AHRQ staff, evaluated all Recovery Act CER contract proposals using the standard criteria that are tailored to the specific needs of each contract solicitation. These criteria include evaluating each proposal's technical approach, management plan, and key personnel. AHRQ officials reported that a contracting officer used the results of the panel's evaluation to make a final selection of contractors that presented the best value to meet the needs of work specified in each Recovery Act CER solicitation.

To meet the September 30, 2010, deadline established by the Recovery Act, AHRQ made one change to its standard contracting process. Specifically, for 1 of the 13 contract solicitations AHRQ conducted an initial review of the contract proposals it received in order to determine whether these contract proposals were duplicative or responsive to the solicitation's requirements.[27] The agency received 23 task order contract proposals in response to this solicitation. Agency officials explained that because they received a large number of proposals in response to this solicitation, they decided to conduct the initial review to identify which of the received proposals would continue through the agency's standard, competitive contract review process. Four of the 23 task order contract proposals were found to be nonresponsive or duplicative of another previously funded study and, therefore, were not considered for further review.

---

[26]When we reviewed AHRQ documentation of out-of-order funding decisions made during the selection of Recovery Act CER grant recipients, we found that although AHRQ officials generally followed the agency's internal policies and procedures to document and review these decisions, the documentation lacked the level of detail required by AHRQ's policies at the time these grants were awarded in 2009 and 2010. The agency revised its policy on the level of detail required to document out-of-order funding decisions on October 3, 2011, to reflect current practices.

[27]This solicitation was for the Evidence Generation priority area.

AHRQ awarded task orders under existing AHRQ master contracts, task orders under existing GSA master contracts, and stand-alone contracts using Recovery Act CER funds. The agency primarily awarded task orders under existing master contracts when awarding contracts with Recovery Act CER funds. Specifically, of the 34 contracts that AHRQ awarded using Recovery Act CER funds, 30 were task orders under either existing AHRQ contracts or existing GSA-schedule contracts, and the remaining 4 were stand-alone contracts. AHRQ awarded multiple task orders within the Evidence Synthesis and Gap Identification priority areas under existing contracts that AHRQ entered into prior to the passage of the Recovery Act. Officials stated that issuing task orders under existing master contracts, which included a GSA-schedule task order, facilitated the quick and efficient award of Recovery Act funds in instances where the agency or GSA had existing master contracts with entities capable of conducting work the agency wanted to support with Recovery Act CER funds.[28] AHRQ officials stated that this approach was faster and more cost-effective than entering into new, stand-alone contracts. AHRQ officials also said that they used stand-alone contracts only in instances where there were existing contracts with entities that could perform the planned work.

AHRQ issued 13 CER contract solicitations between February 2009 and September 2010. Using its standard contracting process and criteria, the agency received 80 contract proposals and entered into 34 contracts totaling almost $161 million.[29,30] These contracts supported HHS's departmentwide and AHRQ's agency-specific CER priorities. (See fig. 3 and app. III for more information on the award of AHRQ's CER contracts with Recovery Act funds.)

---

[28]GAO previously reported that federal agencies primarily awarded Recovery Act funds under existing contracts, such as through task orders. See GAO, *Recovery Act: Contracting Approaches and Oversight Used by Selected Federal Agencies and States*, GAO-10-809 (Washington, D.C.: July 15, 2010).

[29]The 13 contract solicitations issued and 34 CER contracts awarded addressed projects in AHRQ and HHS-departmentwide CER priority areas. Some priority areas were supported by more than one contract solicitation. AHRQ agency-specific and HHS departmentwide priority areas not supported with contracts were supported through grants.

[30]AHRQ made these awards by September 30, 2010, the end of the period in which the Recovery Act funds were available for obligation. See GAO-11-712R. AHRQ awarded an additional $311 million through grants and spent approximately $2 million for administrative purposes.

Figure 3: Distribution of AHRQ's Recovery Act Funds for CER Contracts, by Priority Area

AHRQ's CER priority areas ($98 million total)[a]

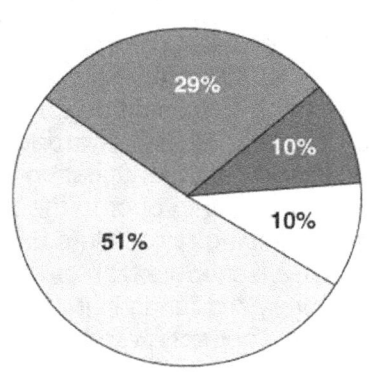

HHS's departmentwide CER priority areas ($63 million total)

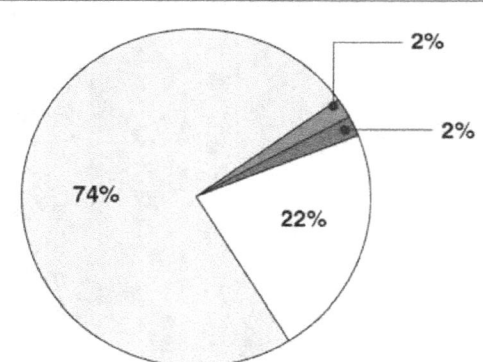

	Percentage[b]	Dollars (in millions)
Horizon Scanning	10%	$9.5
Evidence Synthesis and Evidence Gap Identification	51%	$49.9
Evidence Generation	29%	$28.9
Community Forum	10%	$10

	Percentage[b]	Dollars (in millions)
Data Infrastructure	22%	$13.7
Dissemination and Translation	74%	$46.9
Research	2%	$1.1
Inventory and Evaluation	2%	$1.0

Source: GAO analysis of AHRQ data.

[a]The remaining two of the seven AHRQ priority areas were supported by grants. In addition, contracts awarded for the Evidence Synthesis and Evidence Gap Identification priority areas were combined.

[b]Percentages do not add up to 100 percent due to rounding.

AHRQ Also Reported Taking Steps to Coordinate Recovery Act CER Awards with Other HHS Agencies to Avoid Unnecessary Duplication

AHRQ officials reported that they used five mechanisms in order to coordinate with other HHS agencies to avoid unnecessary duplication when creating FOAs for grants and solicitations for contracts and when awarding Recovery Act CER funds. Specifically, AHRQ participated in a federal interagency coordination council and an HHS working group; contributed to an HHS spending plan to coordinate the department's solicitations; participated with NIH in another working group to coordinate both solicitations and CER awards; and queried HHS databases when awarding Recovery Act funds to identify potentially duplicative projects.

- *Federal Coordinating Council for CER*—AHRQ participated on the Federal Coordinating Council for CER ("the Council"), a body created by the Recovery Act to foster coordination for CER across the federal government in an effort to reduce duplication and encourage the coordinated and complementary use of resources. In addition to AHRQ, officials from the Veterans Health Administration (VHA), the

Department of Defense, and NIH also served on the Council. According to AHRQ officials, the Council provided a mechanism for coordinating, among other things, the establishment of CER priorities and some Recovery Act CER grant announcements and contract solicitations. The Council was terminated by PPACA in March 2010.

- **CER Coordination and Implementation Team (CER-CIT)**—In addition to the Council, AHRQ officials participated in the CER-CIT, a departmentwide effort to coordinate investments in CER supported with Recovery Act funds. Organized by HHS, the CER-CIT served as a centralized forum for HHS officials to assess FOAs for grants and solicitations for contracts. AHRQ officials stated that the CER-CIT's process helped ensure that the FOAs and solicitations ultimately posted by AHRQ for grants and contracts were not duplicative of FOAs and solicitations posted by other entities within HHS. For example, during the CER-CIT's review of two proposed AHRQ CER FOAs, reviewers identified aspects of the proposed announcements that were potentially duplicative of other proposed or existing projects.

- **HHS Intra-Agency Spending Plan**—AHRQ contributed to an intra-agency spending plan developed by HHS that describes how all HHS agencies anticipated using the funding they received under the Recovery Act for CER. AHRQ contributed to this intra-agency spending plan by developing an agency-specific spending plan that described AHRQ's research priorities and how the agency anticipated using its $300 million in Recovery Act CER funds to support these priorities.[31] HHS incorporated AHRQ's spending plan into the department's intra-agency spending plan. According to AHRQ officials, officials from the HHS Office of the Secretary, who were responsible for coordinating this effort, reviewed the spending plans it received from AHRQ and other agencies, and this helped ensure that AHRQ's Recovery Act CER solicitations were not unnecessarily duplicative of other CER efforts within HHS.

- **AHRQ-NIH Working Group**—In addition to the departmentwide working group that was primarily focused on coordination of FOAs and contract solicitations, AHRQ and NIH formed a working group to coordinate the award of Recovery Act funds to avoid unnecessarily

---

[31]Agencies receiving Recovery Act funds were required by the Office of Management and Budget (OMB) to develop a spending plan that documented, among other things, how the agency planned to use its Recovery Act funds.

funding duplicative projects.[32] AHRQ officials stated that before making awards, they checked with NIH through this working group to ensure that the two agencies were not funding duplicative projects. For example, during one meeting members noted where issues of duplication needed to be further discussed to ensure that studies were complementary and not duplicative. In addition to reviewing awards, AHRQ officials reported that this working group met regularly during the award of the Recovery Act CER funds to share spending plans, share solicitations, and provide updates on each agency's respective CER activities.

- **Querying of HHS Databases**—AHRQ officials stated that in order to avoid funding unnecessarily duplicative work with Recovery Act funds, they queried HHS databases prior to awarding any Recovery Act CER funds to ensure that other similar projects were not funded elsewhere within HHS.[33] AHRQ officials stated that if, in the process of querying these databases, a duplicative award was identified, AHRQ would contact the appropriate HHS project officer listed in the database to discuss the award in more detail. AHRQ and NIH officials confirmed that this process resulted in the identification of grant proposals for training awards that were potentially duplicative of projects AHRQ had funded. Once identified, it was decided that NIH would not fund these potentially duplicative awards.

---

[32]According to AHRQ officials, the AHRQ-NIH Working Group is a subcommittee of the NIH Comparative Effectiveness Research Coordinating Committee. AHRQ and NIH are the HHS agencies most active in CER.

[33]According to AHRQ officials, the databases they queried were the Information for Management and Planning Analysis and Coordination II and NIH's Research Portfolio Online Reporting Tools.

AHRQ Plans to Use Its Existing Mechanisms and Develop Additional Strategies to Disseminate CER Results

AHRQ plans to use a range of existing mechanisms, such as written products, training, social media tools, and its website, to disseminate results of CER funded through the Recovery Act. According to AHRQ officials, the agency will determine which specific mechanisms will be used to disseminate CER results by considering the unique characteristics of the research. In addition, AHRQ awarded four contracts using Recovery Act CER funds to develop and implement innovative approaches for disseminating CER results, including Recovery Act-funded CER.

AHRQ Plans to Use a Range of Existing Mechanisms, Such as Written Products, Training, Social Media Tools, and Its Website, to Disseminate Recovery Act CER Results

AHRQ officials stated that the agency plans to use a range of existing mechanisms to disseminate Recovery Act-funded CER results as such results become available. As of December 6, 2011, 30 Recovery Act CER projects were completed or in draft and some dissemination activities had begun.[34] The mechanisms AHRQ plans to use to disseminate Recovery Act-funded CER include written products, training programs, social media tools, learning networks, and AHRQ's website. The different types of written products that AHRQ develops for CER results and other research include comprehensive research reviews that summarize existing research on a CER topic; original research reports that introduce new CER results; and plain language publications that summarize the findings of research on the benefits and harms of different treatment options and which are tailored to clinicians, consumers, or policymakers. AHRQ's training programs include web-based conferences that feature presentations by experts accompanied by instructional slides for clinicians. In addition, the agency employs social media tools to disseminate notices of CER results including electronic newsletters, audio podcasts, and Twitter. AHRQ is also drawing on an existing agency learning network for Medicaid medical directors that was created in 2005. This group convenes periodically to discuss ways to advance the health of Medicaid beneficiaries, including how evidence-based research findings can be used to improve quality of care.[35] AHRQ's website provides access to CER results through search tools and links to its

---

[34]While Recovery Act funds were required to be obligated by September 30, 2010, project end dates may occur after that date. Some projects may take several years to complete and be ready for dissemination by AHRQ.

[35]In addition to this learning network, AHRQ established a learning network that focuses on tools and products related to patient safety.

written and social media formats. (See app. IV for a more detailed description of these existing mechanisms.)

AHRQ officials explained that the agency determines which specific mechanisms will be used to disseminate particular CER results by considering the unique characteristics of the research such as the type of research conducted, its potential impact, the strength of the evidence, and the audiences that can best make use of the information. AHRQ then develops a marketing plan that identifies key messages, target audiences, and the mechanisms to be used to disseminate CER to those audiences. For example, AHRQ's marketing plan for a CER project that examines certain treatments for type 2 diabetes targeted consumers as well as primary care clinicians and certain specialist clinicians and other health professionals. While this CER project was not funded with Recovery Act funds, AHRQ officials confirmed that the process they use to customize the dissemination for this project is the same process the agency will follow for disseminating Recovery Act-funded CER results. To disseminate the CER results of this project to consumers, AHRQ developed a consumer guide and a series of audio podcasts. To reach clinicians, AHRQ developed a clinician's guide and a webcast program with educational slides. These products were targeted to be distributed through multiple channels including AHRQ's website, as well as its newsletters and list-servs. Notices about these products were also sent directly to a range of general media news services; consumer health and advocacy publications; and a wide range of key national organizations that included those representing primary care, specialty clinicians, and payers. (See app. V for a more detailed description of this dissemination effort.)

AHRQ Is Developing Additional Strategies to Disseminate CER Results

In addition to its existing mechanisms for disseminating the results of CER, AHRQ is in the process of developing additional dissemination strategies. Specifically, in September 2010, AHRQ awarded four Recovery Act-funded contracts to develop and implement innovative approaches for disseminating CER results, including Recovery Act-funded CER. The specific purpose of each of the four contracts is described below.

- **Academic Detailing**. Academic detailing involves face-to-face educational sessions by trained clinicians, including physicians, nurses, pharmacists, and others, who visit health professionals in their practice settings. The goal of these sessions is to share evidence-based information and facilitate use of that information to improve patient care. AHRQ awarded a contract in the amount of $11,680,060 for the purpose of implementing academic detailing for CER from 2011 through 2013. The plan under this contract calls for academic detailing to 1,300 primary care providers and 200 health care system practice sites. Each provider or site will receive one face-to-face visit every 6 months plus follow-up e-mail communications and supporting materials. The academic detailing will focus on six CER topics over the 3-year period.[36] Between February 2011 and October 2011, work completed under this contract resulted in over 1,562 visits to providers and practice sites. These visits involved the discussion of AHRQ's CER results related to the treatment of type 2 diabetes.

- **Continuing Education Modules**. AHRQ awarded a contract in the amount of $3,981,168 for the purpose of developing and disseminating 45 accredited online continuing education programs for health care professionals, including physicians, physician assistants, pharmacists, nurses, nurse practitioners, medical assistants, and other health professionals. These programs translate CER results into a variety of formats, for example, videos featuring case studies and journal supplements. As of November 30, 2011, 13 approved continuing education programs were completed, including programs on CER results related to hip fractures, hypertension, prostate cancer, breast cancer, heart disease, and diabetes.

- **Regional Dissemination and Partnership Offices**. AHRQ awarded a contract in the amount of $8,613,876 to create five regional offices for the purpose of establishing partnerships to facilitate dissemination and use of CER results by regional health care organizations, businesses, unions, and consumer groups. Collaborative efforts are expected to result in local and regional meetings, web conferences, training programs, and distribution of CER results to partner organizations' memberships.

---

[36]The first two topics selected for academic detailing under this project address CER related to type 2 diabetes: "Comparative Effectiveness, Safety and Indications of Pre-mixed Insulin Analogues for Adults with Type 2 Diabetes" and "Comparative Effectiveness and Safety of Oral Diabetes Medications for Adults with Type 2 Diabetes." The third topic selected for academic detailing visits is in the area of heart and blood vessel conditions and will be based on the reports titled, "Comparative Effectiveness of Angiotensin-Converting Enzyme Inhibitors, Angiotensin II Receptor Antagonists," and "Direct Renin Inhibitors for Treating Essential Hypertension." As of December 2011 additional topics were expected to cover other heart and blood vessel conditions; muscle, bone, and joint conditions; and/or mental health conditions.

- **Publicity Center**. AHRQ awarded a contract in the amount of $17,999,988 to develop and implement a national strategic communications plan for AHRQ's CER results. The communications plan calls for the development of national partnerships with consumer, clinician, policymaker, and business audiences; marketing efforts, including the use of social media, focused on disseminating results of research; and creation of new website portals with established sites reaching patients and clinicians. For example, under the contract, partnerships have been established with such organizations as the National Rural Health Association, the National Alliance for Caregiving, the American College of Cardiology, and the American Medical Student Association.

Along with its efforts to develop additional strategies for disseminating CER results, AHRQ is taking steps to evaluate the effectiveness of these strategies. Specifically, using its Recovery Act funds AHRQ awarded a contract in the amount of $2,371,179 for the purpose of evaluating some of AHRQ's dissemination strategies by collecting data about dissemination. Under the contract, information will be collected about changes over time in the level of awareness, understanding, use, and perceived benefits of CER . This information will be gathered from clinicians, patients, consumers, health system decision makers, purchasers, and policymakers. In addition, this evaluation includes plans to collect process and outcomes data for each of the additional dissemination strategies being developed under Recovery Act-funded contracts including academic detailing, continuing education, regional dissemination, and the national publicity center.

AHRQ officials noted that evaluating the impact of dissemination of its CER results is important but also challenging. They noted that clinician practice behavior often changes slowly and is affected by many variables, thereby making it difficult to directly attribute changes to information AHRQ has disseminated. In addition, once CER results are disseminated to target audiences through, for example, AHRQ's website or one of its educational programs, it is often not feasible to track secondary dissemination from those audiences to others.

AHRQ Has Begun to Monitor PCORI and Identify Resources That Could Enable It to Fulfill Its PPACA Responsibilities Related to PCORI

While PCORI is in the early stages of development, AHRQ has begun to monitor PCORI's needs to determine what resources might be needed by AHRQ to fulfill its PPACA responsibilities related to PCORI and identify existing resources that the agency can use to fulfill these responsibilities.[37] These responsibilities include broadly disseminating the research findings published by PCORI; developing a publicly available database to collect government-funded evidence and research from public, private, not-for-profit, and academic sources; promoting the timely incorporation of PCORI-generated CER findings into health information technology systems that support clinical decision making; and establishing a process for receiving feedback about the value of information disseminated by AHRQ.[38]

AHRQ officials report that they are monitoring PCORI's needs to determine what resources might be needed by AHRQ to fulfill its PPACA responsibilities related to PCORI. The director of AHRQ serves on PCORI's Board of Governors and another high-level AHRQ official serves on PCORI's methodology committee, which allows AHRQ to obtain information on the resources the institute might need and when these resources might be needed. In addition, according to AHRQ officials, the agency has shared information with PCORI members about AHRQ's existing resources at various PCORI meetings.

AHRQ officials reported that they are also in the process of identifying existing resources, including existing capabilities and ongoing projects, that the agency can leverage to fulfill its responsibilities related to PCORI. For example, AHRQ officials are exploring whether contracts the agency awarded to evaluate AHRQ's CER dissemination efforts could be leveraged to meet the agency's responsibilities to obtain, on behalf of PCORI, feedback from health care professionals on the CER information disseminated by AHRQ. In addition, AHRQ is currently assessing whether a research database being developed by HHS's Office of the Assistant Secretary for Planning and Evaluation could be used to, among other things, store and make publicly available CER funded and generated by PCORI.

---

[37] The Board of Governors for PCORI incorporated the institute in November 2011, and PCORI is in the process of hiring staff to run this nonprofit organization.

[38] See Pub. L. No. 111-148, §§ 6301(a), (b), 10602, 124 Stat. 119, 727-47, 1005 (2010) (to be codified at 42 U.S.C. §§ 299b-37, 1320e).

In addition, AHRQ has developed spending plans for fiscal years 2011 and 2012 that describe how AHRQ will use the funds it receives from PCORTF to fulfill the agency's responsibilities related to PCORI.[39] These plans describe proposed FOAs and contract solicitations that would expand opportunities for AHRQ to disseminate CER information through a variety of channels to different target audiences, for example, public service announcements targeting consumers and symposia and publications targeting researchers and health care professionals. AHRQ officials stated that the fiscal year 2011 plan has been approved by OMB, and the fiscal year 2012 plan was under review by HHS as of December 2011. AHRQ officials stated that they have issued one FOA for a project described in the fiscal year 2011 spending plan but, as of December 2011, have not made any awards.

Agency Comments

We provided a draft of this report to AHRQ for review and comment. AHRQ provided technical comments, which we incorporated where appropriate.

As agreed with your offices, unless you publicly announce the contents of this report earlier, we plan no further distribution until 30 days from the report date. At that time, we will send copies to the Secretary of HHS, interested congressional committees, and others. In addition, the report will be available at no charge on the GAO website at http://www.gao.gov.

---

[39]The funds provided to AHRQ through PCORTF are available until expended. See 26 U.S.C. § 9511(d)(2)(B).

If you or your staffs have questions about this report, please contact me at (202) 512-7114 or at kohnl@gao.gov. Contact points for our Offices of Congressional Relations and Public Affairs may be found on the last page of this report. GAO staff who made key contributions to this report are listed in appendix VI.

Linda T. Kohn
Director, Health Care

Appendix I: The Agency for Healthcare Research and Quality's (AHRQ) Mission, Research, Priorities, and Budget

AHRQ's mission is to improve the quality, safety, efficiency, and effectiveness of health care for all Americans. The purpose of AHRQ's research is to help people make more informed decisions and improve the quality of health care services. AHRQ, formerly known as the Agency for Health Care Policy and Research, is 1 of 12 agencies within the U.S. Department of Health and Human Services (HHS). While the National Institutes of Health focuses on biomedical research to prevent, diagnose, and treat disease and the Centers for Disease Control and Prevention focuses on population health and the role of community-based interventions to improve health, AHRQ's research focus is on long-term and systemwide improvement of health care quality and effectiveness.

AHRQ conducts work in five broad focus areas. These areas include comparing effectiveness of treatments; quality improvement and patient safety; health information technology; prevention and care management; and health care value.

- **Comparing the effectiveness of treatments**. AHRQ's comparative effectiveness research (CER)[1] provides patients and physicians with information on which medical treatments work best for a given condition. This includes comparisons of drugs, medical devices, tests, surgeries, or ways to deliver health care in an effort to help patients and their families understand which treatments work best and how their risks compare. Initiatives under this focus area include:

  - The John M. Eisenberg Center for Clinical Decisions and Communications Sciences

  - Evidence-based Practice Centers

  - The Centers for Education and Research on Therapeutics

  - The Developing Evidence to Inform Decisions about Effectiveness Network

  Quality improvement and patient safety. AHRQ funds and disseminates research that identifies root causes of threats to patient safety, provides information on the scope and impact of medical errors, and examines effective ways to make system-level changes to help prevent errors. Initiatives under this focus area include:

---

[1]AHRQ also refers to CER as patient-centered outcomes research.

- Preventing healthcare-associated infections

- Medical liability reform

- Patient Safety Organizations

- TeamSTEPPS ®

- Patient safety culture assessment tools

- **Health information technology (health IT)**. AHRQ provides support to give access to and encourage the adoption of health IT. The agency has focused its health IT activities on the following three goals:

  - Improve health care decision making

  - Support patient-centered care

  - Improve the quality and safety of medication management

- **Prevention and care management**. AHRQ translates evidence-based knowledge into recommendations for clinical preventative services. AHRQ initiatives under this focus area include:

  - The U.S. Preventative Services Task Force

  - The Patient-Centered Medical Home

  - The Practice-Based Research Network

- **Health care value**. AHRQ aims to find greater value in health care by producing the measures, data, tools, evidence, and strategies that health care organizations, systems, insurers, purchasers, and policymakers need to improve the value and affordability of health care. Initiatives under this focus area include:

  - The Medical Expenditure Panel Survey

  - The Healthcare Cost and Utilization Project

  - Quality Indicators

  - The annual National Healthcare Quality Report and National Healthcare Disparities Report

  - State snapshots

- The Consumer Assessment of Healthcare Providers and Systems

- The National Guideline Clearinghouse

- The National Quality Measures Clearinghouse

In addition to the above focus areas, AHRQ also conducts crosscutting activities related to quality, effectiveness, and efficiency. Activities include data collection and measurement; dissemination and translation; and program evaluation. In addition, support is provided for the investigator-initiated and targeted research grants and contracts that focus on health services research in the areas of quality, effectiveness, and efficiency. These activities provide the core infrastructure used by the other focus areas.

AHRQ staff and budget. AHRQ currently employs approximately 300 staff. The agency's fiscal year 2010 budget was $402.6 million, of which $270.7 million went to research on health costs, quality, and outcomes. The President's fiscal year 2012 budget request for AHRQ was $366.4 million, a decrease of approximately $31 million from fiscal year 2010.[2] (See table 4 for the funding amounts under AHRQ's focus areas.)

---

[2]AHRQ received $369 million for fiscal year 2012 under the Consolidated Appropriations Act, 2012, approximately $2.6 million more than requested. AHRQ's plans for the additional $2.6 million were not yet available at the time we completed our review. In fiscal year 2012, AHRQ will also receive a transfer from the Patient-Centered Outcomes Research Trust Fund (PCORTF) in the amount of $24 million, bringing the total funds available for fiscal year 2012 to $393 million.

Table 4: AHRQ Budget, by Fiscal Year and Research Area

	Fiscal year 2010 Budget (actual)[a] (dollars in millions)	Fiscal year 2012 Budget (President's Budget) (dollars in millions)	Percent change over fiscal year 2010 (+/-)
Research on Health Costs, Quality, and Outcomes (by focus area)			
Patient-centered health research/effective health care	$21.0[b]	$21.6	+2.9
Patient safety	90.59	64.62	-28.7
Health information technology (health IT)	27.65	27.57	-0.3
Prevention and care management	15.9	23.3	+46.5
Health care value	3.73	3.73	0
Crosscutting activities related to quality, effectiveness, and efficiency research	111.79	91.78	-17.9
Subtotal - Research on Health Costs, Quality, and Outcomes	270.7	232.6	-14.07
Other budget line items			
Medical Expenditure Panel Surveys[c]	58.8	59.3	+0.85
Program support[d]	67.6	74.5	+10.21
Prevention and Public Health Fund	5.5	0	-100
Transfer from the Patient-Centered Outcomes Research Trust Fund (PCORTF)[e]	0	24.0	N/A
AHRQ total program level	**$402.6**	**$390.4**	**-3.03**

Source: AHRQ fiscal year 2012 Congressional Budget Justification.

[a]In fiscal year 2011, AHRQ received $372.1 million under the Department of Defense and Full-Year Continuing Appropriations Act, 2011, and $8 million transferred from PCORTF. In fiscal year 2011, AHRQ allocated funds to programs and activities as they had done under the fiscal year 2010 appropriation.

[b]In addition to this amount, AHRQ received $300 million under the American Recovery and Reinvestment Act of 2009 for CER, which was used within this focus area.

[c]The Medical Expenditure Panel Surveys is the only national source for annual data on how Americans use and pay for medical care. The survey collects detailed information from families on access, use, expense, insurance coverage, and quality. Data are disseminated to the public.

[d]The program support budget category supports the strategic direction and overall management of the agency. Program support activities for AHRQ include salaries, travel, rent, supplies, transportation, printing, and other reproduction costs, supplies, equipment, and furniture.

[e]AHRQ receives funding from PCORTF for fiscal year 2011 through fiscal year 2019 to carry out activities outlined by the Patient Protection and Affordable Care Act.

Appendix II: AHRQ CER Grants Awarded Using Recovery Act CER Funds, by Priority Area

Table 5: Grant Applications Received and Reviewed, and Grants Awarded, by AHRQ's CER Priority Areas

Source of Recovery Act funds	AHRQ CER priority area	Number of grant applications received[a]	Number of grant applications submitted for peer review	Number of grants awarded	Amount awarded
Recovery Act Funds Appropriated to AHRQ	Horizon Scanning	0	0	0	0
	Evidence Synthesis	0	0	0	0
	Evidence Gap Identification	0	0	0	0
	Evidence Generation[b]	183	94	19	$148,827,978.00
	Translation and Dissemination	91	49	28	35,670,901.00
	Training and Development	30	26	8	15,384,771.00
	Community Forum	0	0	0	0
	Total	**304**	**169**	**55**	**$199,883,650.00**

Source: GAO analysis of AHRQ data.

[a]The number of grant applications received includes all applications received electronically. Some applications may have been received but not reviewed due to incomplete submission of the application.

[b]AHRQ and the HHS Office of the Secretary jointly funded one grant. For purposes of our report, we counted this grant under the number of grants awarded for the HHS Office of the Secretary's Dissemination and Translation priority area (see table 7). However, the amount of Recovery Act CER funds the HHS Office of the Secretary and AHRQ awarded to this grant are reflected under the amount awarded for the HHS Office of the Secretary's Dissemination and Translation priority area and AHRQ's Evidence Generation priority area.

Table 6: Grant Applications Received and Reviewed, and Grants Awarded, by HHS Departmentwide CER Priority Areas

Source of Recovery Act funds	HHS departmentwide CER priority area	Number of grant applications received[a]	Number of grant applications submitted for peer review	Number of grants awarded	Amount awarded
Recovery Act funds appropriated to the HHS Office of the Secretary and allocated to AHRQ	Data Infrastructure	109	65	39	$77,366,386.00
	Dissemination and Translation[b]	21	´6	6	16,173,967.00
	Research	102	60	10	17,841,781.00
	Inventory and Evaluation	0	0	0	0
	Total	**232**	**141**	**55**	**$111,382,134.00**

Source: GAO analysis of AHRQ data.

[a]The number of grant applications received includes all applications received electronically. Some applications may have been received but not reviewed due to incomplete submission of the application.

[b]AHRQ and the HHS Office of the Secretary jointly funded one grant. For purposes of our report, we counted this grant under the number of grants awarded for the HHS Office of the Secretary's Dissemination and Translation priority area. However, the amount of Recovery Act CER funds the HHS Office of the Secretary and AHRQ awarded to this grant are reflected under the amount awarded for the HHS Office of the Secretary's Dissemination and Translation priority area and AHRQ's Evidence Generation priority area.

Appendix III: AHRQ CER Contracts Awarded Using Recovery Act CER Funds, by Priority Area

Table 7: Contract Proposals Received and Reviewed, and Contracts Awarded, by AHRQ's CER Priority Areas

| Source of Recovery Act funds | AHRQ CER priority area | Number of contract proposals received[a] | Number of contract proposals reviewed | Number of contracts awarded | | | Amount awarded |
				GSA schedule task order	Task orders	Stand alone	
Recovery Act funds appropriated to AHRQ	Horizon Scanning	4	4	0	0	1	$9,499,986.00
	Evidence Synthesis	14	14	0	10	0	49,904,490.00
	Evidence Gap Identification[b]	0	0	0	0	0	0
	Evidence Generation	23	19	0	7	1	28,874,761.00
	Translation and Dissemination	0	0	0	0	0	0
	Training and Development	0	0	0	0	0	0
	Community Forum	9	9	0	0	1	9,999,742.00
	Total	**50**	**46**	**0**	**17**	**3**	**$98,278,979.00**

Source: GAO analysis of AHRQ data.

[a]The number of contract proposals received includes all applications received electronically. Some proposals may have been received but not reviewed for a variety of reasons, including proposals that were incomplete.

[b]AHRQ combined Evidence Synthesis and Gap Identification awards under a single solicitation when announcing the availability of these funds and within awards because, according to agency officials, having a single solicitation for these two priority areas reduced the amount of work related to these awards, thereby expediting the award process. As a result, AHRQ funded both of these priority areas, but advertised projects and made awards for these priority areas under a single solicitation.

Table 8: Contract Proposals Received and Reviewed, and Contracts Awarded, by HHS Departmentwide CER Priority Areas

Source of Recovery Act funds	HHS departmentwide CER priority areas	Number of contract proposals received[a]	Number of contract proposals reviewed	Number of contracts awarded			Amount awarded
				GSA schedule task order	Task orders	Stand alone	
Recovery Act funds appropriated to the HHS Office of the Secretary and allocated to AHRQ	Data Infrastructure	11	11	0	4	1	$13,683,264.00
	Dissemination and Translation	15	15	4	2	0	46,856,206.00
	Research	2	2	0	1	0	1,060,353.00
	Inventory and Evaluation	2	2	0	2	0	1,008,456.00
	Total	**30**	**30**	**4**	**9**	**1**	**$62,608,279.00**

Source: GAO analysis of AHRQ data.

[a]The number of contract proposals received includes all applications received electronically. Some proposals may have been received but not reviewed for a variety of reasons, including proposals that were incomplete.

Appendix IV: AHRQ Mechanisms That Support Dissemination of CER

Types of mechanisms supporting dissemination	Examples of AHRQ's dissemination mechanisms
Written products	• Research reviews and original research reports: These written products draw on completed scientific studies to make comparisons of different health care interventions or summarize original clinical research to explore practical questions about the effectiveness of treatments. • Summary treatment guides for clinicians, consumers, policymakers: Short, plain-language guides summarize the findings of research reviews on the benefits and harms of different treatment options. • Education modules and presentation slides: These resources are for clinicians pursuing continuing education credits and for faculty who are instructing clinicians.
Training programs	• Webcasts: Researchers and clinicians participate in online programs to discuss research findings. • Conference series: Scientific meetings on state-of-the art concepts in communication, health literacy, and medical decision making.
Social media tools	• Audio podcasts: The Healthcare 411 audio podcast series shares news and information with consumers that they can use in health care decision making, through 60-second audio news programs and longer format interviews. • Online videos: AHRQHealthTV provides videos for consumers about a range of health topics on AHRQ's YouTube channel. • Twitter updates: Short messages are broadcast that can be accessed by computer or mobile phone. • RSS Feeds: Subscribers receive news and alerts about AHRQ programs through their RSS reader. • E-mail updates: Subscribers receive e-mail updates on topics they are interested in.
Learning networks and case studies	• The Medicaid Medical Directors Learning Network: This is one example of a network formed by AHRQ to create an ongoing collaborative relationship to disseminate AHRQ products, tools, and research to help members make policy and practice decisions related to clinical treatment. • Impact Case Studies: AHRQ tracks and summarizes how AHRQ-funded research, tools, and products are actually implemented by state governments, medical practices, clinics, and hospitals. Makes summary information available to other potential users.
Website and other resources	• AHRQ's website ahrq.gov provides access to its written products, training programs, and social media tools, as well as useful search functions and other resources. • Health Care Innovations Exchange: The Exchange offers health professionals and researchers searchable tools to access information about evidence-based innovations suitable for a range of health care settings and populations, as well as opportunities to network with other professionals who have implemented these innovations.

Source: AHRQ.

CER topic	Comparative Effectiveness and Safety of Premixed Insulin Analogues in Type 2 Diabetes: A Systematic Review
Background	Type 2 diabetes is an increasingly common chronic disease that occurs in people who have too much glucose in their blood. Blood glucose levels are high either because their cells are resistant to insulin (a hormone that helps convert glucose into energy) or because their pancreas does not produce enough insulin. Insulin analogues are used approximately as commonly as human insulin by diabetics who require insulin to regulate blood glucose levels. Created by genetically modifying human proteins, insulin analogues were developed as an alternative to human insulin to provide tighter control of blood sugar levels.
Key findings	This study summarizes the effectiveness of insulin analogues against traditional human insulin for type 2 diabetics. Researchers compared the effectiveness of three kinds of synthetic insulin against their human insulin counterparts, against each other, and against other antidiabetic medications. The report found that insulin analogues are more effective than human insulin for treating certain diabetes-related symptoms such as high blood sugar after meals. However, it also found that human insulin appears to be more effective than insulin analogues in treating other aspects of diabetes, including lowering blood sugar levels when patients go 8 hours or more without eating, typically overnight.
Products and formats	<ul><li>Press release</li><li>Comparative effectiveness report</li><li>Executive summary</li></ul> <ul><li>Consumer guide (for adults)</li><li>Clinician's guide</li><li>Webcast and slides (for clinicians)</li><li>Audio podcast (for consumers)</li></ul>
Key audiences	Over 90 target organizations, publications, and electronic venues are identified in the marketing plan in the following categories: clinicians, insurers, payers, pharmacy and drugs associations, federal direct and funded medical care programs, consumer-oriented disease organizations, and government. Provider categories targeted include retail and health system pharmacists; family physicians and general internists; pharmacologists; nurse practitioners; physician assistants; and endocrinologists.
Media outreach	General media news services including radio, television news, and major daily newspapers; consumer and advocacy publications; African-American media; and translation to Spanish-only and Hispanic media.
Other electronic targets	Medscape, WebMD, ModernMedicine.com, ePocrates
AHRQ publications	Electronic Newsletter, Effective Health Care Listserv, Research Activities newsletter, Website Spotlight

Source: AHRQ.

Appendix VI: GAO Contact and Staff Acknowledgments

GAO Contact	Linda T. Kohn, (202) 512-7114 or kohnl@gao.gov
Staff Acknowledgments	In addition to the contact named above, E. Anne Laffoon, Assistant Director; Shaunessye Curry; Mary Giffin; Andrea E. Richardson; Lisa Motley; Krister Friday; and Jessica C. Smith made key contributions to this report.

GAO's Mission	The Government Accountability Office, the audit, evaluation, and investigative arm of Congress, exists to support Congress in meeting its constitutional responsibilities and to help improve the performance and accountability of the federal government for the American people. GAO examines the use of public funds; evaluates federal programs and policies; and provides analyses, recommendations, and other assistance to help Congress make informed oversight, policy, and funding decisions. GAO's commitment to good government is reflected in its core values of accountability, integrity, and reliability.
Obtaining Copies of GAO Reports and Testimony	The fastest and easiest way to obtain copies of GAO documents at no cost is through GAO's website (www.gao.gov). Each weekday afternoon, GAO posts on its website newly released reports, testimony, and correspondence. To have GAO e-mail you a list of newly posted products, go to www.gao.gov and select "E-mail Updates."
Order by Phone	The price of each GAO publication reflects GAO's actual cost of production and distribution and depends on the number of pages in the publication and whether the publication is printed in color or black and white. Pricing and ordering information is posted on GAO's website, http://www.gao.gov/ordering.htm. Place orders by calling (202) 512-6000, toll free (866) 801-7077, or TDD (202) 512-2537. Orders may be paid for using American Express, Discover Card, MasterCard, Visa, check, or money order. Call for additional information.
Connect with GAO	Connect with GAO on Facebook, Flickr, Twitter, and YouTube. Subscribe to our RSS Feeds or E-mail Updates. Listen to our Podcasts. Visit GAO on the web at www.gao.gov.
To Report Fraud, Waste, and Abuse in Federal Programs	Contact: Website: www.gao.gov/fraudnet/fraudnet.htm E-mail: fraudnet@gao.gov Automated answering system: (800) 424-5454 or (202) 512-7470
Congressional Relations	Katherine Siggerud, Managing Director, siggerudk@gao.gov, (202) 512-4400, U.S. Government Accountability Office, 441 G Street NW, Room 7125, Washington, DC 20548
Public Affairs	Chuck Young, Managing Director, youngc1@gao.gov, (202) 512-4800 U.S. Government Accountability Office, 441 G Street NW, Room 7149 Washington, DC 20548